SPICA
SUPERHEROES

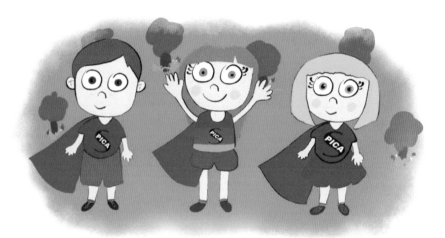

Written by:

KAREN KERR

Illustrations by:
Mina MacDougall

My Daughter,

Lauren Kerr

My true inspiration and the one who kept me
going through
it all.

A true Spica Superhero

Xxx

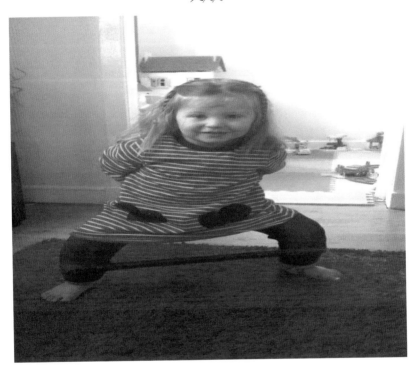

I call her name.

I like to call patients into clinic myself. It seems more gentle, more human, more polite. It means I can watch them walking before they know that that is what I am watching.

She brings her family with her - Mum and Dad and Gran: this bold, smiling just-two-year-old. And as she bowls towards me, with her big tummy, and swaying from side to side, I pretty much know the conversation we will be having over the next hour: I will be outlining an uncertain sequence of operations and Spica casts that are going to dominate their lives for the next 6 months. And beyond.

Even before I examine her, I know that she doesn't have a big tummy, rather a very arched back pushing the tummy forwards – it's just the 'tummy' we see. And she has the very arched back to compensate for the fixed flexion at her two dislocated hips. She sways side-to-side, her pelvis dipping on one stance side, then the other. It's a characteristic pattern: a 'Trendelenburg' gait.

Trendelenburg was one of the German forefathers of surgery, a man who studied here at Glasgow a century and a half ago, about 400 meters away from where we are in clinic. As we are sitting and talking, Gran tells me, 'She walks just like my mam, when my mam was old and had arthritis'. That's one of the things about 'Trendelenburg': it applies across the lifespan, albeit for different reasons.

Later we talk through the X-rays. With the pictures I can show what's really wrong. The X-rays make it clear, definite - parents know they have a problem. I talk slowly, methodically, and for quite a while, hopefully gently. (Outside the waiting-room is noisy, and Anne, our outpatient nurse, will be writing a number by my name indicating how late the clinic is running – (so that people know'). This appointment is going to take as long as it takes – certainly rather longer than the 15 minutes templated. Like in the operating-theatre, the patient in front of you is the focus, the one that matters.

I talk about DDH, about its spectrum for problems, about what would happen if we did nothing, about what our common aim might be, about how to get there, about the risks their beautiful daughter is running by having treatment; a treatment that will involve a sequence of operations – open reductions both hips, bilateral femoral osteotomies, bilateral pelvic osteotomies, multiple scars, and extended immobilisation in a Spica. We talk about the risks of disturbing the blood supply to the femoral head, changing its shape, avascular necrosis, re-dislocation, pressure sores and infection. We talk about the actual percentages.

We talk about the far future, about their daughter as a young woman, about pain now for deferred gain: hopefully, all being well.

After all this, I bring up the 'Trust's 'time-to-treatment guarantee', how with my operating waiting-list being what it is, I can arrange transfer to one of my colleagues, if they desire, or else they can waive TTG stipulation to stay under my care. Although 'targets' are set up with good intentions, they have some bizarre unintended consequences. I am only too aware of the inappropriateness of applying targets from the adult sector to children, and also of having this conversation as a tag-on. They stay with me.

I take them to the plaster room, to meet one of our fantastic technicians. Alison will take some time, with photos, models and dolls to go through what a Spica is like, about car chairs and high chairs, and about the practical parts of living with a Spica, everything a family needs to know. Our plaster team are upbeat, understanding, capable and empowering. They give courage, and parents need that.

Five operations, however many Spicas, and five years on... now I see her once a year, maybe for ten minutes: my privilege and snapshot of a smiling youngster growing up. She has an X-ray, and I examine her hips.

So far, every time is an improvement, all is well.

Jim Huntley March 2017
James Huntley
MA MCh DPhil MB BChir MRCSEd
FRCSGlas FRCPEdin FRCSEd (Tr&Oth)
Paediatric Orthopaedic Consultant Surgeon,
RHC, GlasgoHonorary Clinical Associate
Professor & Barclay Lecturer,
University of Glasgow

Lauren's x-ray pictures, before and after clearly showing why the legend Mr Huntley was worth waiting for (Karen Kerr)

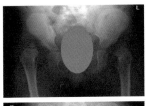

2 years age

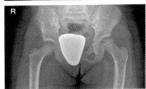

6 years age

Such a special thanks to Mr Huntley for the emotional foreword
(Karen Kerr, Grant Kerr and Lauren Kerr)

Introduction

Hi, we're Lauren and Lucas, we're the Spica Superheroes. We both have hip dysplasia and have spent lots of time in a Spica cast.

We are here to look after other girls and boys just like us.

You can be a Spica Superhero too!

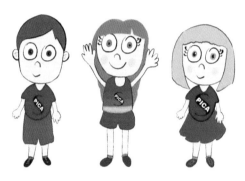

Diagnosis

We want you to meet our friend Hollie.
Hollie is 3 years old and loves dancing and gymnastics, unfortunately she's just been told she has hip dysplasia.

Hip dysplasia is where the leg does not fit into your hip socket a bit like a ball in a cup.

Hollie is upset and scared as she knows she will need an operation to fix her hip and must spend time in a Spica cast.

A Spica cast is like special hard trousers that you wear all the time that keeps your hip in place.

We have explained that the operation won't be scary. She will be asleep the whole time

The Doctors will take excellent care of her and her Mummy and Daddy will be there when she wakes up.

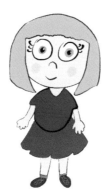

Preparation for operation

It's not long now Hollie until you must go into hospital to have your operation.

Your Mummy has bought you a table called a Spica table which you can sit at while you have your cast on. This means you have a place to draw, do your jigsaws and eat. She has also got you some lovely dresses to wear while in your cast as it is very difficult to fit clothes over the cast.

The Spica table will be very good to help you sit and play as it will be difficult to move around when you have the cast on. This doesn't have to be a bad thing though! You get to sit at your table all day doing jigsaws, drawings, watching TV, or if you're really lucky playing iPad! Remember Lauren and I are here if you are worried before you go in to hospital!

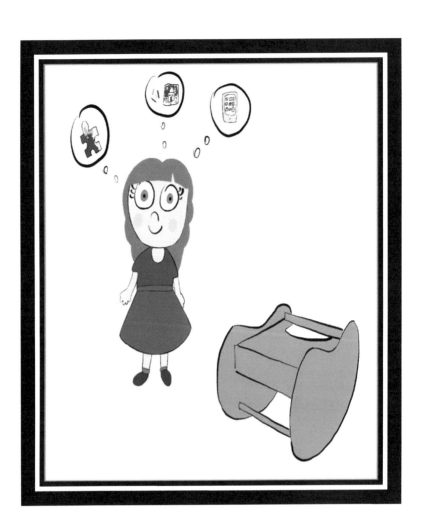

Morning of operation

On the day of the operation you must get up quite early to go to hospital.

You won't be able to have any breakfast but when you wake up after the operation you will be able to eat and drink.

When you get to the ward at the hospital the nurse will show you to your bed. She will give you a wrist band with your name on it so everyone knows who you are.

Then the doctor will come speak to you and check you over to make sure you are well enough to have your operation. They will draw an arrow on the leg that they will be doing the operation on. You will then get to jump into bed and wait until It is your turn to go. When it's your turn you get to stay in bed and you get driven to the theatre. To have your operation you must be asleep. To do this they ask you to wear a mask that blows out air which makes you sleepy.

Before you know it, you're sleeping!! Your' Mummy or Daddy will be with you the whole time!

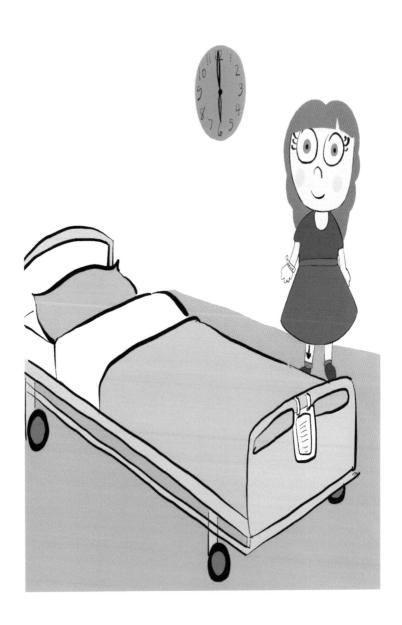

Post operation

When you wake up from your sleep you will have your "new legs" we spoke about. It will feel strange at first as you can't move around much. You will quickly get used to your new Spica cast and learn ways of getting around!

You might also feel a bit sore and uncomfortable but don't worry the nurses will look after you. They will give you medicine to help your pain go away.

Lastly you must be thirsty and hungry because you didn't have breakfast. Your throat might be a bit sore when you wake so drinking lots will make you feel better.

It is important to drink lots after you have an operation but I'm sure you can do this for Lucas and me!!

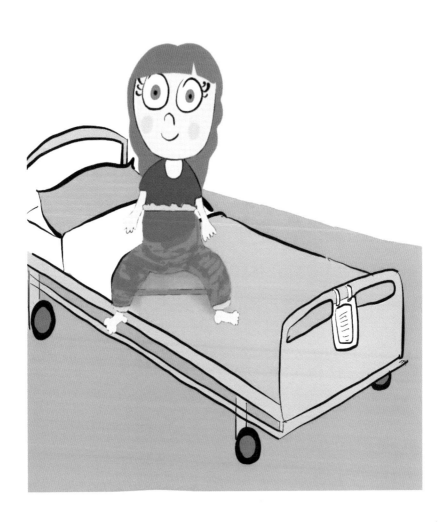

Time in hospital

Hi Hollie, Lauren and I wanted to come visit you and see how you were getting on with your new fancy pink legs! When Lauren was in her Spica cast that was her favourite colour too.

Your Spica will take you a bit of time to get used to but once you're home you'll find your own way of doing things and no doubt getting around!

You're going to be in hospital for another day or so for the doctor to make sure you are well enough to get home. While you are waiting to get home a special nurse called a plaster nurse will visit you and your Mum.

This nurse will teach you how to look after the cast at home and what to do if any damage happens to it. She will also explain that you can call her at any time if have any worries about the Spica cast.

Soon you will be home and you will get to show everyone your shiny and tough new pink legs!

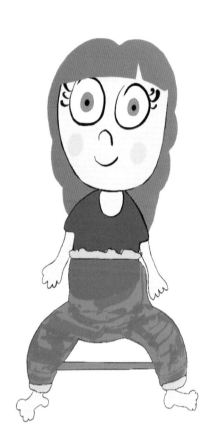

At Home

Lauren and I heard you were out of hospital and wanted to see how you were getting on. You look as if you are all organised with your beanbag, Spica table, jigsaws and iPad!

I also see you're getting around a bit in your cast by crawling.
This will get easier for you the longer you are home, do keep at it!

I wanted to tell you in a few weeks' time you must go back to hospital to have a new Spica cast put on. Please don't worry as there is no operation this time so no pain and you will only be in hospital for the day and be back home by teatime.

So, in the meantime you keep practicing getting faster round the floor. Your' Mum won't be able to catch you soon!!

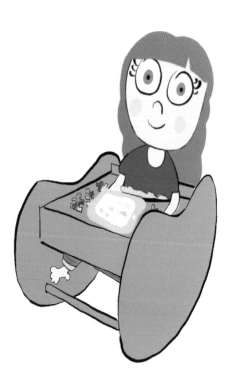

Cast change

Lauren and I wanted to come with you while you got your cast changed today.
The cast you have on just now will be getting very dirty and a bit loose so you will need a new cast on to last you for the final weeks.
Don't worry though this time is much easier than when you had your operation.
You won't be in pain this time and you will get to go home on the same day!
It's also the last step before we have legs again!
YAY!

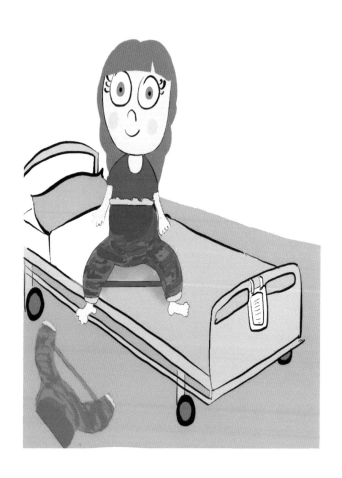

Cast off/ Spica Superhero

Hollie it's time to get your cast off!
It's going to be noisy but please don't worry
it won't hurt.
They use a set of cutters to open the cast which
are very noisy but again not sore.
You can close your eyes when they start, and
when the noise has stopped open your eyes and
you will see your legs again!

Not only that because you have been through
this Spica journey you have become a Spica
Superhero too!!

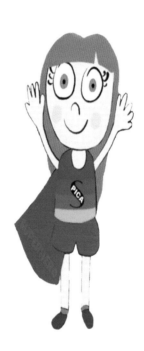

About Me,

My name is Karen Kerr. My Spica Superhero is Lauren.

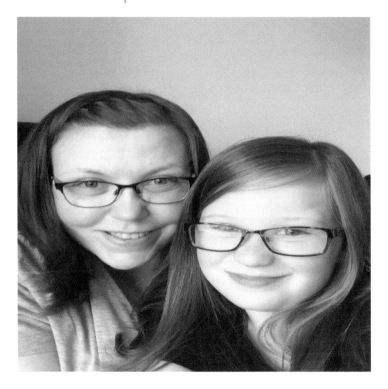

I am, I guess now an author, good one or otherwise remains to be seen. Please feel free to let me know @ karenkerr@live.co.uk

I wrote this book for several reasons, the main one being to help you, your partner and

MOST importantly your little Spica Superhero.

You are unsure of what to expect I imagine, you have doubts, fear, worries and questions. Thankfully there is resources, my book and in the world of social media Facebook groups to allay and answer all the above. Shout out to "DDH UK HIP DYSPLASIA SUPPORT GROUP"

I am a Mum of a Spica Superhero, a braver, more determined and independent girl you will never meet, Lauren, my daughter suffered from bi – lateral hip dysplasia and spent 18 months in a cast and not a thing stopped her, let me tell you. Jeez at times I wish it had, she walked, climbed, jumped and excelled whilst in her cast all despite 6 serious operations.

You know what, your little one will do much the same. They are an inspiration and a true reflection of each of us as parents, be proud. That's an order!

I would like to thank a few people for getting me to where
I am today. Some of these people are fellow parents, some not, some are personal friends and some I have met along the way

Dot Kerr – my husband's mum and the rock who listened when we were too emotional to, she has been there and reassured us as parents from birth and continues to now.

Debbie Favell – Canadas newest immigrant

and a true friend despite never meeting her,

her words of encouragement have assisted me

in getting to where I am, when doubts have

crept in she has booted my

"hin' end" and told me to get on with it. A

taskmaster second to none. She cares for me,

checks on me and has proof read and

encouraged me to complete this project.

Mina Mcdougall for picking up this as a

project, for your unfaltering support and

illustrations for the book, you have been there

since I can remember for me and have stepped

up to the mark yet again. A debt I shall

never repay except maybe in pizza, coffee

and possibly babysitting.

Natalie Trice – she has a page to herself so I won't
go on too much about her but she knows she has
been there when I have needed her.

Ashley and Hollie

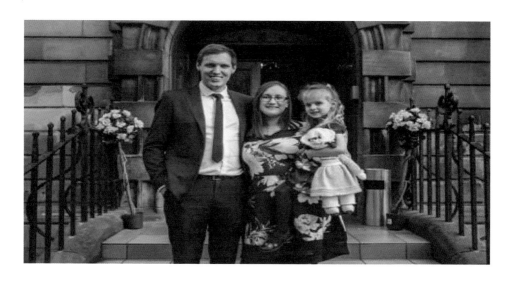

Our journey: after going to see several doctors and physio, at
22months Hollie was eventually sent for an X-ray and was confirmed having DDH in her left hip.
About 6 weeks later, just
after her 2nd birthday she was having surgery to try and correct it.
Hollie spent 12 weeks in a Spica cast. She has had a long recovery, attending physio for several months.

Hollie would have really benefited from a book like this to help her understand what was going to happen, as I was not fully aware of what was involved.

Acknowledgement

I would like to take a minute, if I may to recognise another resource and to some degree inspiration, both for mums of cast kids but for
me. Natalie Trice is a freelance blogger and author and without her I feel I would never have had the courage and determination to write this.

Her book,

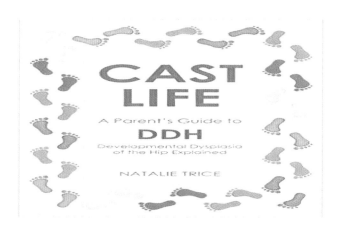

This is a great aid in many a cast kid and Spica parents journey I am sure. Through networking and discussions my book has come to fruition. I would like to share a few words from Natalie herself. Please feel free to purchase Natalie's book as an additional resource to aid in your cast journey where the talented author shares a vast plethora of opinions and experiences from herself and other parents,